The Wellness CAPSULES

LITTLE PELLETS OF HEALTH AND GOODNESS

SUJATA NAIK

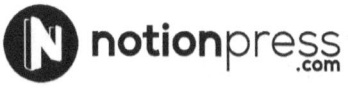

INDIA • SINGAPORE • MALAYSIA

Notion Press

Old No. 38, New No. 6
McNichols Road, Chetpet
Chennai - 600 031

First Published by Notion Press 2019
Copyright © Sujata Naik 2019
All Rights Reserved.

ISBN 978-1-64587-920-6

This book has been published with all efforts taken to make the material error-free after the consent of the author. However, the author and the publisher do not assume and hereby disclaim any liability to any party for any loss, damage, or disruption caused by errors or omissions, whether such errors or omissions result from negligence, accident, or any other cause.

While every effort has been made to avoid any mistake or omission, this publication is being sold on the condition and understanding that neither the author nor the publishers or printers would be liable in any manner to any person by reason of any mistake or omission in this publication or for any action taken or omitted to be taken or advice rendered or accepted on the basis of this work. For any defect in printing or binding the publishers will be liable only to replace the defective copy by another copy of this work then available.

Disclaimer: The Wellness Capsules is not a medical text, nor meant to substitute expert opinion in anyway. It is an attempt to draw attention to common place, yet uncommon perception of little, yet significant aspects of life that can be connected to health and wellness in any way. It has been a random collection of some loud thoughts aimed at the reader, to ponder and get inspired.

For every person who considers health and wellness a personal responsibility

Contents

Preface 11
Acknowledgements 13

1. A Capsule with a Difference 15
2. Space from Discipline 16
3. Letting Go 16
4. Smile Please 17
5. Angry Rash 18
6. Virtually True 18
7. Quick Start for a Day 19
8. Go, Bid 20
9. Good Nights 20
10. Pain in the Neck 21
11. Swish 22
12. Fighting Fatigue 23
13. Squat to Stay Fit 24
14. Sore Muscle? 24
15. Thought Shower 25
16. A Good Massage 26
17. Get the Door 26
18. Cool Buttermilk 27
19. Mouth Going Dry 28
20. Think Today 29
21. Brew Trouble 29

22.	Go Guava	30
23.	Strike and Pocket	30
24.	Figure Yoga	31
25.	Stay in Love	32
26.	Bless You, Sneeze	33
27.	Smelly Feet	34
28.	Happy Emotions	35
29.	Posture Relief	36
30.	Edgy Nails	36
31.	Inner Invests	37
32.	Tense Moments	38
33.	Wellness Gyaan	39
34.	An Egg Everyday	40
35.	Jet Lagged?	41
36.	Air-Borne Gut	41
37.	Rising Sun	42
38.	Alternative Binging	43
39.	A Cooler Summer	44
40.	Foresight	45
41.	Glowing Skin	46
42.	Ageing Gracefully	46
43.	Clear Nose	47
44.	Double Deal	48
45.	Beware the Anticlimax	49
46.	Happy Gut	50
47.	Smart Weekends	50
48.	Gift Away	51
49.	Love Heals	52
50.	Honest Policy	52

51. Body, Mind, Soul 53
52. Crying Releases 53
53. Small Wins 54
54. Smelling Sense 55
55. National Immunity 56
56. Voting for Wellness 56
57. Budgeting for Health 57
58. Sleepless? 58
59. Super Monday 59
60. Fresh and Fine 59
61. Watch Your Back 60
62. Friends for Therapy 61
63. Hung Curd Option 62
64. Dignity of Labour 63
65. Golden Silence 63
66. Travellers' Travails 64
67. Hic Hic 65
68. Wellness Shots 66
69. Practising Patience 66
70. Squeaky Clean 67
71. Super Shoes 68
72. Knead Away 68
73. In Emergencies 69
74. Through Chemotherapy 70
75. Chill Pill 71
76. Ordinarily Special 72
77. Working Nights? 73
78. Cut Down the AC 74
79. Cashing on Food 75

#	Title	Page
80.	Long Drive	76
81.	A Healthy Liver	77
82.	Salt Free	78
83.	Steer Clear of Virus	79
84.	Supplements for Immunity?	80
85.	Haandvo Meal	80
86.	Telltale Signs	81
87.	Up the Defences	82
88.	Doing Nothing	83
89.	Natural Dryer	83
90.	Gossip Therapy	84
91.	Spacing Out	85
92.	Weathering the Bone	86
93.	Working Long	87
94.	Jaggery for Dessert	88
95.	Goodness Good?	89
96.	Pampered Gut	90
97.	Help for Mental Health	91
98.	Skin Tags	92
99.	Colour You Choose	93
100.	Red, Blue…and Green	93
101.	*Ganne* Ka Ras	94
102.	Stomp Away	95
103.	The Warrior's Family	96
104.	Sleep in the Dark	97
105.	Train the Tremor	97
106.	The Crisp Newspaper	98
107.	Nurse the Caregiver	99
108.	Visible Calories	100

109.	One Two Ka Two	100
110.	Watch the Blood Sugar	101
111.	Overcoming Personal Loss	102
112.	Moisturize Your Lips	103
113.	Extra Sleepy?	104
114.	Chalk, Clay and Cheese	105
115.	That Sprained Ankle	106
116.	Waiting for the Burp	107
117.	Unto Wellness	107
118.	Nurture the Girl Child	108
119.	Vitamin *Amla*	109
120.	Cleanliness Home-delivered	110
121.	Pray, for Wellness	111
122.	Do Your Homework	112
123.	Whose Life is it Anyway?	113
124.	Strumming Fingers	114
125.	Mind your Fingers	114
126.	Phantom Pain	115
127.	Plug That Leak	116
128.	Simple Fasting Rules	117
129.	Razor Sharp	118
130.	Move on, Failure	118
131.	The Road Less Taken	119
132.	Water Tales	119
133.	Starving a Fever	120
134.	Hair Where?	121
135.	Only 99?	122
136.	Road Rage	123
137.	Hearing in Style	124

Contents

138. A Pinch of Salt 125
139. Shoulder Freeze 126
140. Throw Away the Toxins 127
141. Your Doctor – Your Soldier 128
142. The Unbeatable *Khichadi* 129
143. Tough Back 130
144. *Anna Purnabrahma* 131
145. Think Abundance 132
146. Springing the Pet Pack 133
147. That Pain! 134
148. Strengthen That Shyness 134
149. Herb Garden 135
150. Greying Prematurely 136
151. Thinning Eyebrows 137
152. The Powerful Om 138
153. Stretch the Stiffness 139
154. An Eye for the Eyes 140
155. Flying Ankles 141
156. The 3 am Confidants 142
157. Healthy Investment 143
158. Blocked Ears? 144
159. Raw *Kairi* 145

About the Author *147*

Preface

The unexpected and overwhelming response to my first publication, 'The Wellness Shots' – a compilation of my health and wellness tips on social media, spruced up my enthusiasm and confidence to write the next. The continuing demand for my health posts pushed me to start this new series. While this has also been connected to health and wellness, it is different from the earlier format. 'The Wellness Capsules' are little, power-packed doses containing my own perception, based on more than three decades of clinical practice, of anything that could be connected with health and well being. Be it physical or mental, it is the small, positive corrections in daily living that could go a long way in promoting and maintaining wellness. As a health care provider, one's responsibility goes far beyond treating disease and managing ill health; patient education and social awareness regarding truths and myths about lifestyle, diet and disease ought to be a major mission too. If these little capsules have succeeded in cheering up and encouraging even the slightest shift towards healthy living in the reader, I consider my task largely accomplished!

Acknowledgements

Writing a book and all the labour and insecurities that go with it, is like childbirth; the pain forgotten once the baby is out. The second delivery was a tad easier with the experience of the previous book 'The Wellness Shots' still fresh. Having my consultant and dear friend, Gayathri Thakoor, by my side, my clinic team ready with every errand, and the continuing support of Notion Press has provided a huge level of comfort, which cannot be overemphasized. The meat of the credit for 'The Wellness Capsules' belongs to each of my thousands of patients who have encouraged and inspired me with their faith and trust, and to all the readers who followed my daily clinical tips on social media, to egg me on to come out with an extension of my earlier work. No creative work, big or small, can ever be possible without a behind the scenes backup! I am blessed to have such an understanding family that is so magnanimous in putting up with phases of neglect from me on the home front, during the peak working stages of this book. I am also hugely grateful to young Zai Thakoor, who has through her pictorial illustrations and creative capabilities added brightness to the capsules.

A Capsule with a Difference

The medicinal capsule is made up of an outer gel and polysaccharide coating to dissolve at the right time after reaching the stomach. The contents are the medicinal ingredients which are released into the bloodstream at the opportune time for maximum absorption.

The Wellness Capsule is made up of an outer cover, that of our body constitution which conceals and protects our core constitution. The contents of the capsule include our innate immunity which needs to be used at the right time in right proportion for maximum benefit.

The medicinal capsule fights disease, the Wellness Capsule protects health!

What would you rather take?

Space from Discipline

An important key to wellness is to allow yourself flexibility – in diet, exercise, sleep, and even punctuality! Self-discipline to the point of rigidity may release stress hormones resulting in exactly the opposite of what one is trying to achieve!

Letting Go

The forgetful may rejoice.

Those who forget, forgive and let go, have been observed to have an active prefrontal cortex (the part of the brain controlling emotions), thus enjoying better neurological health.

So, stop trying to remember, instead let's learn to forget!

Smile Please

A smile adds to much more than just face value. Even when forced, a smile can reduce blood pressure, elevate mood and improve it. Practise smiling at everyone you meet, when on the phone or even when you don't feel like it. It will still improve the levels of positive hormones.

For the naturally nasty, fake it until you can make it!

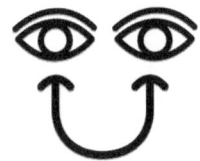

Angry Rash

To get relief from prickly heat rash, wear fully covered, light and loose cotton garments which can help evaporate sweat from the skin. Apply the juice of grated cucumber and Aloe vera over the rash, along with 5 drops of Urtica Urens 200c (available at any local homeopathy pharmacy) taken with 1 tbsf of water, twice a day. It may reduce the irritation and inflammation to a large extent. Above all, keep cool. *An angry skin is a reflection of a disorder within!*

Virtually True

Social media is the greatest communicator and the greatest alienator too! Virtual relationships may lead to serious loneliness and depression. To keep your relationships going in the real world, *sometimes do switch off the internet and press the CALL button!*

Quick Start for a Day

Grouchy and grumpy in the morning? Some suggestions to spruce up your wake time:

* Get up before 7am no matter what time you may have gone to bed.
* Do not lie in bed for even a few minutes after waking.
* Music of your choice is great to get your spirits up.
* Have a shower within minutes of waking up as a quick kick start to the day.
* Plan at least one pleasurable activity for the next day at bedtime – meeting a friend, a movie, a dinner or even a good book.
* Smile at the cranky face in your mirror, a guaranteed smile in return!

Go, Bid

A game of cards everyday is the best way to delay dementia. For the elderly, it is an excellent bridge of communication, *an effective way of making them feel included and loved!*

Good Nights

Incontinence and increased frequency of urine especially at night can be a nuisance for the elderly. Once underlying major conditions are ruled out, encourage the use of diapers. *A little added cost after initial inhibition are certainly worth a good night's sleep!*

Pain in the Neck

Have a pain in your neck? Not always an orthopedic issue, it could be neurological! A good GP who knows your health history and predisposition sends you to the right specialist who can fix it. *Let your family doctor be your first point of contact.* Always!

Swish

The typical Indian tradition of rinsing one's mouth immediately after a meal is proven to be one of the best methods to maintain oral hygiene. Brushing right after eating may harm the enamel whereas rinsing thoroughly can dislodge the food particles between the teeth gaps and remove at least 30 per cent of the bacteria Adding a pinch of cinnamon powder to the rinse will be a wonderful mouth freshener too! Whether at home, a wayside eatery or a fine dine place, this simple ritual following every meal is bound to *reduce your visits to the dentist!*

Fighting Fatigue

Tiredness is largely a physical symptom related to exhaustion from overwork or inadequate sleep and certain medical conditions that include deficiencies, diabetes or cardiovascular disease. A correction of the underlying cause helps. Fatigue, on the other hand, is a persistent low-energy symptom coupled with loss of motivation which needs psychosomatic evaluation. *Time to visit a homeopath!*

Squat to Stay Fit

To be able to squat well into your sixties indicates excellent muscular and neurological fitness and the secret of a good bowel movement too. Indian toilets involve squatting and should certainly be encouraged. Western commodes could be reserved for the old, infirm and arthritic!

Sore Muscle?

For all the marathon runners suffering from muscle soreness and joint aches, a few doses of *homeopathic Arnica 30c* followed by *Rhus Tox 30c* will keep you in ship shape!

Thought Shower

Need an instant mood lift? Sing in the shower! Bathroom singing reduces cortisol – the stress hormone, improves lung capacity, boosts confidence and may even bring an extra glow to your face. At no cost. Just a little perhaps, *a cortisol rise in the person on the other side of the door!*

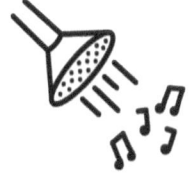

A Good Massage

Regular massage helps to stimulate blood circulation to muscles, increasing their flexibility. It can also release toxins and help tone up muscles making you appear slim. Does massage actually help to shed weight? Yes, of course, that of the masseur!

Get the Door

Most cardiovascular episodes are sudden and happen at night. For all 60 years and above, or even younger with hypertension or diabetes, *Never lock the bathroom door.*

Cool Buttermilk

Buttermilk, truly an elixir of life, is a very affordable, low calorie drink packed with vitamins and minerals and is ideally made with one part of yogurt and 9 parts of water. It is a cooling, carminative drink, tolerated by every age and the lactose-sensitive too. Have it with a pinch of cumin, rock salt and asafoetida … and rest assured, *the skin will not erupt, the stomach will not rumble and your pocket will not grumble!*

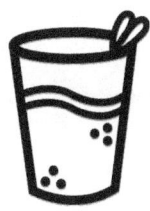

Mouth Going Dry

Persistent dryness of mouth especially at night and the need to wake up in between to sip water, is probably a symptom of obstructive sleep apnea, typical of mouth breathers. Rule out anemia, diabetes and deficiency of Vit B12 too. Sucking on unsweetened amla (gooseberry) candies, avoiding table salt and drinking enough water is the solution. At bedtime, rinse your mouth thoroughly with a mug of warm water and squeezed lime, avoid medicated mouth washes and menthol lozenges, and preferably sleep on your sides. This will ensure that your mouth will not go dry except when asking the special one out on a date!

Think Today

Someday, most of us would lose the ability to walk, to pee, to reason. How does one prepare to minimise suffering in that phase of life? By eating well and eating right, by remaining active at whatever age, inculcating healthy habits, building a healthy bank balance and investing in deep, happy relationships. When is the right time to start? *It was yesterday!*

Brew Trouble

A beer belly is not just a sign of prosperity, it's an invitation to hernia. How does one prevent one? Eat smaller meals, have enough fibre to get regular bowel movement, chew food longer, do regular yoga and have walks, cut down on aerated drinks and *of course, beer!*

Go Guava

It's not an apple a day … it's a guava a day that keeps the doctor away. A guava is richer than an apple in antioxidants, vitamin C and dietary fibre … ideal for *diabetics, weightwatchers, the constipated and the cost-conscious!*

Strike and Pocket

Carrom is one of the best board games as it is enjoyable, played in a group and improves both visual perception and brain body coordination. Exchange the fancy digital games for this *wonderful, underrated and yet so affordable Carrom!*

Figure Yoga

In a nation with cultural, environmental and economic diversity, is there something that can improve the stamina, immunity and wellbeing of its citizens at zero cost? No prizes for guessing… If every Indian gave only half an hour of the day to Yoga, the national productivity would go up by 200 per cent. *Wellness does not need expensive equipment, just a resolve!*

Stay in Love

Falling in Love is a transient phase associated with a rush of adrenaline and cortisol making it heady and exciting but stressful, whereas Staying in Love is linked to secretion of dopamine and serotonin, making it a calm, happy stress-relieving phase. This Valentine's Day, *choose to Stay in Love!*

Bless You, Sneeze

The old wives' tale about a sneeze during a severe illness being a good omen is actually true. Occasional, minor illnesses like acute colds, coughs and fevers tease the immunity into gearing itself for a potential major attack, thus strengthening it. So the next time you have a cold or a fever, do not pop a pill to suppress it. Rather, take a day off from work *to allow the body to service itself!*

Smelly Feet

To combat foot odor in warm, humid months, wash feet and dry thoroughly, especially between the webs of toes where bacteria thrive. Dust Calendula powder on the inside of the shoe. Wear socks made from thin mixed fabric. Thick cotton socks may absorb moisture and get smelly. Change socks twice daily and shoes every alternate day. The spare pair should hang out to dry in the sun – *the best disinfectant in the world!*

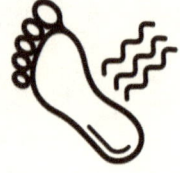

Happy Emotions

Negative emotions can have adverse impact on psychological and physical health. Amongst them, malice is easily the most toxic! An intense, deep-seated ill feeling towards someone, malice can damage the rational thinking of the one harbouring it and the self-confidence of the one aimed at. When it persists, it may be instrumental in eroding one's constitution and may act as a trigger for serious medical conditions. Good emotions can be cultivated. Replace malice with empathy, gratitude and benevolence, *and see the remarkable positive contribution to your health!*

Posture Relief

Prolonged standing and sitting may result in tired, aching feet, swollen ankles and varicose veins. Weight control, sitting with feet raised and compression stockings may help. Aesculus 30c, one of the several useful remedies in homeopathy for varicose veins, will certainly give relief from the tortuous trouble!

Edgy Nails

To get out of the annoying habit of nail biting, try chewing sugarless gum, wearing gloves or simply applying gel paint to nails, making it difficult to chew them off! Begin by addressing the root cause – whether anemia, anxiety or boredom!

Inner Invests

Importance of good quality inner garments is often overlooked. Avoid silk and synthetic, damp, ill-fitting undergarments; use only soft, pure hosiery cotton. This will protect you from various fungal infections, and some potentially serious ones! Put off the external finery, *first invest in inners!*

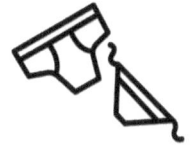

Tense Moments

When facing viva exams, job interviews or competitive tests on public platforms, performance anxiety may result in acid reflux and an embarrassing desire to keep clearing the throat of mucus. Avoid milk-based beverages, fatty foods, aerated drinks, fruit juices, or even a meal at least two hours before the event. A few sips of plain water and a dose of homeopathic Argentum nitricum 30c will help reduce nervousness *to help you come out with flying colours!*

Wellness Gyaan

Some quick mantras for total health and wellness:

- Eat less, chew more.
- Sit less, walk more.
- Stand less, sleep more.
- Pluck less, plant more.
- Frown less, smile more.
- Brood less, think more.
- Envy less, appreciate more.
- Talk less, do more.
- Text less, talk more!

An Egg Everyday

This one is for eggetarians. Children, weight watchers, cholesterol watchers, diabetics, and even those with a history of heart disease, you may safely have the entire egg. Do not discard the yolk, as it contains the best stuff of the egg including its iron, folate and vitamins. The next time when the white is eaten and the yolk becomes the hair conditioner, remember … *your hair is what you eat and not what you apply!*

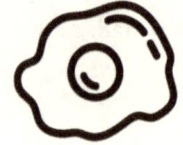

Jet Lagged?

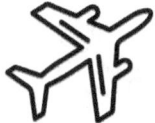

The best way to prevent jet lag is to stay hydrated, eat little, keep moving and convert to the current time zone. Still groggy? Try Cocculus indicus 30c. *Just a couple of doses should set you right!*

Air-Borne Gut

Frequent air travel against time zones may disturb the digestive function leading to bloating and upset bowels. Increasing water intake, reducing alcohol, having regular but light meals, along with homeopathic remedy Mag mur 30c taken for a couple of days, could ease gut dryness. *Aconite 30c may relieve bathroom anxiety in alien toilets!*

Rising Sun

Watching the sunrise is a tremendous energy booster and mood elevator, particularly beneficial for arthritis and asthma. The first rays of the morning sun bring in a soft, radiant light exuding hope and positivity. Besides, free for all, no taxes! The only problem – one needs to wake up when the sun does!

Alternative Binging

Lazing and binging over the weekend after slogging through the week can be more stress-inducing, causing serious fluctuations in your metabolism. Instead, snatch moments of leisure during a packed week and plan activities during weekends. A surefire stress buster … a short, brisk walk followed by a relaxed snacky meal at your favourite restaurant on a Wednesday evening … *It's possible, check it out today!*

A Cooler Summer

Summer brings on the heat and sweat, yet the sensation of internal heat and burning could also be due to anxiety, stress, hormonal imbalance or certain medication. Drinking water at regular intervals, eating watery fruits like pineapples, oranges and watermelons to replenish the lost electrolytes, and having a bath with lukewarm water could help reduce internal heat and burning. Basil seeds or *sabja* soaked in water and taken with some cold milk are great internal coolers. If burning persists, *a few doses of Ars alb 30 taken over a couple of days can help!*

Foresight

Sometimes, just a progressive disinterest in studies without other symptoms should alert a vigilant mother to rule out shortsightedness in her child. Early correction with appropriate glasses is the only way to treat myopia. Pushing carrot and pumpkin juice down the poor child's gullet will not reverse it. Healthy eating with sufficient greens should be inculcated from the mother's pregnancy itself. It is the parents' vision which determines the child's too. *Pun absolutely intended!*

Glowing Skin

Not all fairness creams are harmful, if used with discretion. Note however, that they have bleaching and anti-tan effects which only give an illusion of fairness. They cannot make a sick skin glow. A skin that radiates glow is the one that reflects healthy living and a happy constitution … whether white, brown or ebony!

Ageing Gracefully

Botox and anti-ageing creams may remove superficial signs of ageing, a few wrinkles and some skin tags. What can really keep you youthful long beyond your chronological age is happiness that radiates from within: a reflection of years of good health, self discipline and inner calm … the extra glow from living for a larger social cause!

Clear Nose

A dry, stuffy nose disturbing sleep is common during winter months. A quick shower at bedtime with warm and not hot water, followed by a 3–5 minute steam inhalation with a few Eucalyptus leaves infused water and a few pills of homeopathic remedy Arum triphyllum 30c for a couple of days *should bring beauty back into your sleep!*

Double Deal

For a change, try using your non-dominant hand (eg. the left hand if you are right-handed) for simple tasks like picking up your cup, pouring water from a jug, using the computer mouse, combing your hair or even brushing your teeth. Not as simple as it sounds, yet training to become ambidextrous is like teasing the brain and shaking it out of its complacency to becoming more creative. *A harmless adventure at no extra cost!*

Beware the Anticlimax

The dream success after years of hard work can be surprisingly anticlimactic. The high levels of cortisol that keep up energy levels during planning and working may fall flat as soon as the objective is achieved, leading to a low, empty phase, perhaps depression too. The remedy? Keep moving! Engage in physical exercise and recreation to recuperate your adrenaline for the next goal. Be forewarned – *the greater the success, the greater may be the anticlimax!*

Happy Gut

Do not overdo the health diet by excess intake of fruit, greens, whole grains and raw sprouts. Too much fibre could lead to indigestible matter clogging your intestines, increasing fermentation and worsening constipation. Gut health depends on balance between soluble and insoluble fibre. *Only a healthy gut reflects a healthy constitution!*

Smart Weekends

To avoid weekends becoming cheat days, sleep in late, head straight for a late lunch, eat your fill, have a 20-minute nap, go for a 45-minute brisk walk and have only steamed sweet potatoes for dinner. *This way you have your cake and save it too!*

Gift Away

Try this today – Gift away something you bought for yourself. The joy and gratification on the face of the receiver and the release from your own attachment will result in a surge of the 'feel good' hormone serotonin *in both; a little more in the giver!*

Love Heals

True love can never hurt, it can only heal. Love can reduce the stress hormone cortisol, up the positive hormone dopamine and actually release natural opioids, which can minimise pain. To treat ill effects of unrequited, misunderstood, misplaced love, *there is homeopathy!*

Honest Policy

Honesty is not just truthfulness, it is about being real with yourself and others too. Being honest in every action increases confidence, strengthens willpower and improves vitality. It is a quality that can minimise stress, improve relationships and keep you well. *Honestly*!

Body, Mind, Soul

Physical fitness alone is not a guarantee of wellness! Just as the best instrument will play the perfect tune only if the skill, focus and soul of the player are in rhythm, one will experience total health only if the body, mind and soul are in perfect harmony!

Crying Releases

It's not only laughter that is the best medicine. Crying can be therapeutic too. Emotional crying is a great cleanser as tears release toxins, chemicals, dust and debris along with endorphins, the natural painkillers. Laughter energizes, crying catharizes. *Laugh to feel good, cry to feel better!*

Small Wins

Celebrating even small successes can boost well being. It can instill confidence in the team set out for a bigger goal. Every little accomplishment celebrated with close ones is a motivator, a rejuvenator, and most importantly, takes the stress off the final task. Never wait for the Big Win ... the fun, the adrenaline is in the anticipation – *a reward for now and an incentive for later!*

Smelling Sense

Diminished or absent sense of smell (anosmia) is largely due to sinus congestion from recurrent cold or following a brain injury. Pulsatilla 30c, if taken for a couple of days, and a saline nasal wash may reduce congestion and restore the sense of smell. Anosmia is a very distressing symptom as it takes away flavour from food which depends both on the taste buds and olfactory sense. Feel blessed whenever you smell your favourite curry! *Not everyone is so lucky!*

National Immunity

In a national crisis whether natural, political or security, every citizen should avoid panic, maintain calm and offer constructive help. Performing duty and avoiding mass hysteria are huge contributions. Let the individual strength of each citizen help build the collective immunity of the nation!

Voting for Wellness

Individual health is linked to community health which in turn is linked to national health, which is totally dependent on good governance. Only a strong, stable government elected through a healthy mandate can moot and implement health policies sensitive to the citizens' needs. This is how precious that single vote is. It determines your health, perhaps even your lifespan!

Budgeting for Health

10 per cent of every family's income must be dedicated to a health budget which should cover:

1) a contingency fund for medical emergencies
2) regular medical expenses
3) a good medical insurance package.

Never needed the insurance? Well, it's not money wasted, it is health earned!

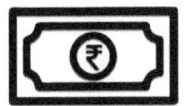

Sleepless?

Tired, but cannot sleep? Tiredness may not result in sleepiness. If one gets into bed without feeling sleepy, insomnia is likely to occur. Too much excitement, stimulants or intense mental work before bedtime result in sleeplessness. Although physically tired, if your mind is racing or crowded with thoughts, sleep may elude you. In such a situation, one dose of homeopathic Coffea cruda 6x may settle that restless, overactive state to put you into snooze mode.

Super Monday

The best way to kickstart your week is to wake up a few minutes early, do a 5-minute intense exercise, munch a fruit for breakfast, dress your best and get to work fifteen minutes earlier than usual. *A stress-free Monday sets the tone for the week!*

Fresh and Fine

How do you know you have slept enough? It could be as less as five hours and as much as eight hours. What matters is if you fall asleep within ten minutes of getting into bed, wake up feeling rested and refreshed and do not need to nap during the day, you are blessed with one of the most vital parameters of Wellness!

Watch Your Back

Much of our back health depends on the choice of the mattress. A bad mattress can ruin the back and sleep. The right mattress must be firm, not hard … soft, but not wobbly. Individual preference and adaptability can vary greatly; therefore, always buy the mattress after a trial of at least 48 hours. One secret though, the peaceful sleeper will sleep on rock and the insomniac will toss and turn. The poor mattress will continue to be at the receiving end of the blame!

Friends for Therapy

Our immune system can deal with an acute injury or infection. It is the chronic, morbid diseases that induce maximum suffering. For those suffering from diseases like debilitating arthritis, chronic asthma, Parkinson's or Psoriasis, the challenge is to get over the disease by making the best of the situation. Apart from good nutrition and physical activity, a few true, non-judgmental, empathetic friends … and most of all, those who encourage you to look at the lighter side of life are, in fact, perhaps your real therapy!

Hung Curd Option

For cheese lovers on a low sodium, low calorie diet, hung curd blended with pepper, rock salt and crushed mint can be a nutritious, equally tasty substitute. Line a roti made from ragi flour with the hung curd mixture, and roll to make a unique, wholesome wrap!

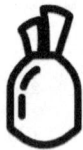

Dignity of Labour

Everybody as a matter of habit must make one's own bed and wash one's own toilet! How is that linked to wellness? Doing the above improves hygiene, encourages activity and inculcates dignity of labour. The melting of ego in the process is tremendously therapeutic. *Begin today!*

Golden Silence

Go on a verbal diet once a week! Silence helps increase sensitivity to other body functions, improves focus and lessens the toxins entering our body. If an entire 'non-speaking' day seems impractical, spend an hour of total silence, while minimising the rest of the day's conversations. *If nothing, peace is guaranteed for your spouse!*

Travellers' Travails

A big source of distress and embarrassment is the traveller's diarrhea. When on the go, persons with sensitive digestion should rather stick to well-cooked bland food and avoid rich food, meat and dairy products (except tea/coffee with very little milk). Bottled drinks though higher in sugar are to be preferred over fresh juice as they are unlikely to induce infection. Most diarrheas are self-limiting, and maintaining fluid and salt balance is important. Even if on a day trip, carry a packet of oral rehydrating solution … and yes, an extra set of clothes too!

Hic Hic

Hiccups are harmless, irritating diaphragmatic spasms and are generally self-limiting. If holding one's breath, swallowing cold water or eating sugar do not help, sipping ice water very quickly through a straw and taking a dose of Carbo veg 30 are effective remedies. If the hiccups do not stop for over 48 hours, your doctor will rule out other causes. *If you are an alcoholic, a hiccup is a dead giveaway!*

Wellness Shots

Stress from a financial setback can be a harbinger of cardiovascular ailments, insomnia, depression and hormonal fluctuations. During this, keep away from escape routes like smoking, alcohol or excess eating. This is the time to invest in what money cannot buy – *healthy habits, forgotten hobbies and true friendships!*

Practising Patience

Patience is a virtue that has multiple health benefits. Persons who are innately patient have slower pulse rates, lower blood pressure and are more optimistic. To practise patience, let go of the need of instant gratification and learn to wait a bit before you react. A few successful attempts at waiting before reaching for your favourite dessert could actually help you get over the craving. *It's all about winning over that one moment!*

Squeaky Clean

Clean hands are the best mode to prevent diseases like diarrhea, dysentery, typhoid and jaundice (infective hepatitis). However, avoid sanitizers where water and soap are available. Instead, distribute the sanitizers and encourage their use in slums and areas with poor access to sanitation. It will be your contribution to community wellness and *Swachh Bharat*!

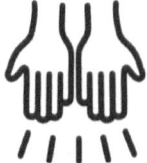

Super Shoes

Choose your footwear with care, the focus being comfort first, style later! Ill-fitting shoes can disturb the alignment of the entire spine resulting in tired, aching feet that are bad enough to ruin your entire day. The best test of good shoes is being able to *forget you are wearing them!*

Knead Away

Kneading and rolling dough to make rotis is a great exercise for the shoulders, arms and small joints of the hand. It can significantly reduce stiffness associated with early arthritis, keep muscles supple and improve peripheral circulation. *This is one kitchen chore one would rather not give up!*

In Emergencies

With the elderly, cardiac patients, diabetics, hypertensives or those with chronic ailments in the family, it is best to prepare a synopsis of the patient's health history, predispositions or history of allergies, if any, and attach it to the medical records for quick reference – to help in sudden emergencies!

Through Chemotherapy

Cancer patients on chemotherapy may suffer from intense nausea and distaste for food during treatment. Frequent bites of dry cereal, toast, roasted nuts, salted snacks, dry roasted papads, sugar coated cookies and chilled juice should help. Avoid your favourite foods at this time; these may be the ones you may not want to look at. Homeopathic remedy Colchicum 200 could help reduce persistent nausea and food aversion. Good nutrition is the most vital factor in sustaining cancer treatment!

Chill Pill

Unexplained irritability, depression and low energy levels without any obvious physical ailment could indicate an underlying disease. Time for a chill pill! Rest, relax and see your doctor. A disturbed constitution sends subtle signals before pathology manifests. Nip the problem at the outset to bounce back with renewed vitality!

Ordinarily Special

When the monotony of daily, ordinary routine bogs you down, ask the paralyzed how special it is to be able to hold that cup of coffee, the handicapped what it means to walk, the cancer-stricken undergoing chemotherapy what it means to have a normal appetite or the Alzheimer's patient how extraordinary it is to remember one's own name. If you enjoy normal health and appetite and lead an active and independent existence, feel blessed; *it is only the special who are blessed to be ordinary!*

Working Nights?

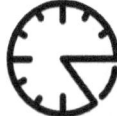

The 3 am to 5 am time slot is the toughest for those on night shifts. Munching fatty, salty snacks and caffeine to keep awake will add unhealthy calories and disturb the biorhythm. Unsalted nuts, fruit, or a low sugar protein bar along with sipping warm water with basil, lemon grass and honey helps staying up bright through those crucial duty hours!

Cut Down the AC

To prevent premature wrinkling, keep the use of air conditioner to the minimum: it blocks sweat pores and reduces natural hydration. Activities that trigger breaking into a sweat help in opening up skin pores, keeping it supple – A few minutes of brisk walking, for instance, *or perhaps your wife checking your phone!*

Cashing on Food

If the diet you are on – whether all carbs or no carbs – is keeping you thinking about food all the time, you've got it wrong! Money and food contribute to wellness only when you have enough. How much is really enough? *Money in your pocket, food in your stomach, neither in your head!*

Long Drive

Some suggestions when leaving on a self-driven trip and to keep the spirits and energy up …

- Get adequate sleep before and after the drive
- Avoid alcohol at least 24 hours before travel
- Munch roasted snacks – roasted papads are excellent
- Sip masala chai during halts

Sniffing from a spray of a strong scent like citrus or eucalyptus intermittently *will help prevent dozing off at the wheel!*

A Healthy Liver

Our liver takes the maximum responsibility of practically every metabolic process in the body. It is the first organ to handle stress and the last to give up, making us being able to survive with even just one third of it. So treat your liver with respect. Plenty of fruit, green vegetables, sprouts, whole grains, fresh juice, tea, coffee and fresh air are all liver-friendly. Alcohol, tobacco, rich greasy food, meat and processed food are to be taken sparingly and selectively. So, what does the health of the liver really depend on? *Of course, the liver!*

Salt Free

Going for a party tomorrow, want perfect pictures but looking bloated? Do not skip meals. It will make you look wilted. Instead, have regular meals, only go salt free. Also sipping lemon squeezed in water every few hours will draw the excess sodium from the cells making you look fresh and trim ... *just right for all those selfies!*

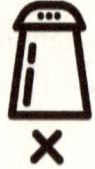

Steer Clear of Virus

The sudden fluctuation in temperature increases transmission of viruses through air and contact. The solution:

- Adequate clothing to cover chest, neck and ears
- Drink enough water
- Wash hands more often
- Avoid closed public places (auditoriums, malls)

And, for a few days no hugs, only 'Namaste'!

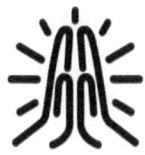

Supplements for Immunity?

Simple, fresh food, good sleep, enough sunshine, and an active, cheerful disposition are all that is required to boost one's immunity. Nutritional supplements should be reserved for post infection debility and those with proven deficiencies. Excess of these will get excreted *and fatten the rodents in the sanitary drains!*

Haandvo Meal

If you are looking for a wholesome, delicious complete one-dish meal, try the Gujarati *Haandvo*! A fermented and baked combination of rice and various lentils with generous portions of vegetables, greens and a tempering with mustard and sesame packs it with every nutrient, *thus qualifying its place in a midday school meal or even at fast food counters!*

Telltale Signs

Nature has gifted the human body with a wonderful immunological defense that tries to tackle a disease at the superficial level, before it can attack a vital organ: an itch, a rash, recurrent boils, mouth ulcers, sudden unexplained hair loss, a sore or cut that refuses to heal, sudden appearance of warts or any outgrowths that could be a sign of an impending illness. *Never ignore, never suppress!*

Up the Defences

Just as a country prepares itself for war by fortifying its defences during peace time, one's body too must prepare for a potential terror attack, read disease, during good health. Adequate diet, exercise, sleep, enough sunshine, work satisfaction and happy relationships together strengthen the immune system for use, when the body is under stress. Be prepared always ... *Note that the enemy will invade only if the ground is weak!*

Doing Nothing

So much to do and cannot get yourself to do it? Simple. Do Nothing. Doing nothing at the peak of stress is an art and has tremendous health benefits. It brings the stressed body to zero gear, ups the dopamine, reduces the cortisol *and fuels up for the battle ahead!*

Natural Dryer

Drying washed clothes outside in the sun is not unclassy, it's totally hygienic. The UV rays of the sun are free, natural sanitizers, aborting bacterial and fungal growth on clothes, drying them completely and making them smell fresh. Whenever possible, choose the sun over machine dryers, *your clothes will last longer too!*

Gossip Therapy

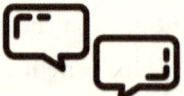

Gossip, if harmless, can be an easy conversation starter, an outlet for introverts and a great therapy for stressed souls! A fun talk of others' real/ imagined personal affairs gives a vicarious pleasure, like adding spice to a bland meal. Of course, it's only a myth that it's the women who enjoy gossip. *Try eavesdropping into a men's locker room!*

Spacing Out

Modern lifestyle often contributes to brain fog, affecting mental clarity and concentration with a cloudy feeling during the day. Check to see whether you are overstressed, are not getting enough sleep, or suffer from B12 deficiency or a thyroid issue. Light meals and long walks are a sure shot for a remedy. Still need help? Take Acid phos 12c twice a day for two weeks *to clear the cobwebs from your brain.*

Weathering the Bone

Once the joints are worn and torn, the damage is practically irreversible. Creaking joints, a laughable possibility in the twenties, becomes a reality in the fifties and even the early forties. Weight control, aerobic exercise, a diet rich in calcium, Vitamin C and protein, and adequate rest should be inculcated early to preserve bone health in later years. Those crazy outdoor games in the blazing hot sun do better for your immunity and bones than *the artificially pumped Vit D and calcium supplements!*

Working Long

Work life balance is important for wellness yet not always linked to work hours. Six hours of work can tire you while a 12-hour workday can still keep you in high spirits! The key is to enjoy your work, make time for some open-air exercise, regular water breaks at work (not junk/coffee ones), a few minutes for laughter and an uninterrupted sleep! Hard work kills no one. *It's stress from an unfavourable work environment that is the killer!*

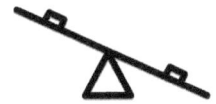

Jaggery for Dessert

A small lemon-sized piece of jaggery at the end of your meal is a healthy substitute to any dessert and will effectively reduce your craving too. Jaggery contains some amounts of iron and potassium and is a natural way to combat iron deficiency. Surprisingly, it can aid digestion due to its fibre content. The dark, unprocessed one got from molasses is the best. *A no-no for diabetics and moderation for the rest!*

Goodness Good?

It's not only bad habits and vices that predispose to illness. Teetotalers, non-smokers and extremely conscientious, duty driven individuals often succumb to disease as they have not provided their bodies the rest and recreation it may have required to build immunity. Nature seeks balance to provide longevity. *Extreme goodness too may shorten life span!*

Pampered Gut

Evacuating one's bowels thrice a day or thrice a week –
there is really no normal parameter. It is the satisfaction
with your motions that is important. Habitual laxatives,
stool softeners and enemas can damage the lining of the
intestines, best avoided. The obsession with evacuating at
a certain time everyday induces stress, causing constipation
on the rebound. Report any unusual pain, bloating
or sudden change in bowel movement to your doctor.
Otherwise, learn to be happy with your gut!

Help for Mental Health

Depression is an unexplained, persistent low mood. If under depression, never fake happiness or normalcy. Accepting the problem, coming to terms with it and seeking help is the first step to cure. Also, depression is often associated with loneliness and isolation. Indulging in group activities with physical exercise may help. Note that depression is not a phase ... it's a malady of the mind that calls for medical help. *It may happen to the best of us!*

Skin Tags

A middle age cosmetic nuisance – skin tags – are little, unsightly growths on the neck, face and folds of skin. They could also indicate hypothyroidism, high cholesterol, obesity, diabetes and insulin resistance. Check first if any of the above apply to you. A homeopath can offer you effective remedies, and a dermatologist can cauterize them. If the skin growths don't irritate, embarrass or bother you, *they're best left alone!*

Colour You Choose

Heads up to green, the colour of nature, healing, fertility and abundance. Whatever is green, edible and natural is packed with vitamins and minerals, and builds immunity leading one to Wellness. Tails down to green, the colour of jealousy, ambition and greed – all destructive emotions! The choice is yours. *Which side of the coin you flip!!!*

Red, Blue…and Green

During busy working hours, spare a few minutes to look out of the window to focus your eyes on any patch of greenery. Trees and plants emit oxygen, energy and positivity. Just looking at the colour green can soothe tired eyes that are irritated from the blue of electronic screens. A quick walk on the green grass is even better … *only if your boss does not see red!*

Ganne Ka Ras

Treat your guests to a refreshing glass of sugarcane juice. Sweeter than sweetened juices yet lower in glycemic index, it's an excellent oral rehydrating drink during fevers, urinary infections and stomach disorders. If constipated, a glass of fresh sugarcane juice daily will get your bowels moving!

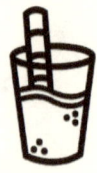

Stomp Away

This one is for our soldiers, policemen, home guards ... the stomping during parades may cause overuse injuries or even fractures at vulnerable sites including shin bones. Ruta 30c to hasten healing and Calcarea fluoricum 30c as strengthener for ligaments and bones, taken twice a day for a couple of weeks along with conventional measures, are safe and effective homeopathic remedies to protect those who guard us!

The Warrior's Family

The aftermath of a war tragedy can inflict shock and may result in long lasting post-traumatic stress in the soldier's family or in the witnesses to the incident. Let us reach out to those affected by offering counselling, moral support and medication. It is not enough to grieve for the dead, *it's more important to care for the living!*

Sleep in the Dark

Always sleep in complete darkness as the hormone melatonin which regulates sleep, is secreted only in the dark and never in any artificial light. Lack of melatonin predisposes to obesity, hence refrain from use of even the softest night lamps. Wild animals never stay up beyond sunset. *Hence they never need to deal with weight gain!*

Train the Tremor

Involuntary shaking of the head, hand and voice (essential tremors) is common and mostly harmless among the elderly. Reassurance, physiotherapy and anxiolytics are generally prescribed. If either of the parents has suffered from the above, one is likely to inherit it. Start weight training today, one of the best preventions for essential tremors!

The Crisp Newspaper

Reading a newspaper daily improves focus, increases general knowledge and language skills, and widens one's horizons. The e-newspaper, while providing similar information, encourages surfing and browsing resulting in reduced attention span and must be discouraged. The habit of reading the newspaper daily is the best window to knowledge and self-confidence and must start from childhood. *Some traditions are best continued!*

Nurse the Caregiver

With professional nursing care, being unaffordable to most, looking after a terminally ill or bed-confined elder can be stressful to even the closest family member. Take turns with other well-wishers to relieve the caregiver by attending to the patient at least for a few hours. *The goodwill earned by this noble gesture will be beyond measure!*

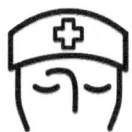

Take a pause today to thank the most vital caregiver in a patient's journey to recovery – the Nurse! Someone who works as hard, is as dedicated and certainly more compassionate to the patient's suffering than a doctor, and deserves more prestige and better material rewards. For, it is perhaps only a nurse who is indispensible in the first and last moments of human life!

Visible Calories

If you are on a diet check, note this. During social meals, eating only a bite of every dish from the huge spread is, in fact, adding invisible calories and deluding you into believing you have eaten less. Rather, stick to one favourite dish and have it to your heart's content. *And now compare the calories!*

One Two Ka Two

The daily tradition of recitation of mathematical tables, writing a page to practise handwriting and being read out bedtime stories remain some of time's tested rituals for children to enhance creativity, memory and motor skills! Stronger parent-child bonding is an added benefit. *Can the best gadget in the world replace that?*

Watch the Blood Sugar

Diabetics beware! Never juggle with your medication or stop it abruptly. Fluctuations in blood sugar levels could cause irreparable damage to the kidney, heart and brain. All the lifestyle and dietary corrections may reverse the prediabetic phase and help prevent complications in a diabetes patient, yet cannot replace the existing medication in an established diabetic. *The corrective measures should have been taken before you got there!*

Overcoming Personal Loss

Devastated may it be, the human body still has an amazing capacity to bounce back to normalcy after bereavement following a loved one's loss. In extra-sensitive, introvert individuals, the grief may be unnatural, prolonged and bottled up. Such persons will do well with a few doses of homeopathic remedy Ignatia. *What time cannot heal, homeopathy will!*

Moisturize Your Lips

If dry, flaky lips persist, after ruling out dehydration, vitamin deficiencies, allergies, auto-immune skin conditions or drug reactions, try this simple remedy. Take a mixture of 1 tsf sugar, cream of milk and 15 drops of Calendula tincture, and rub over the lips twice daily. *Sugar will exfoliate, cream will moisturize and Calendula will heal!*

Extra Sleepy?

If you feel excessively sleepy during the day after your usual night-time quota, do consider a thyroid check. An underactive thyroid gland is responsible for lower concentration, lethargy and sluggishness, with low productivity at work. Very often, symptoms are subtle and start much earlier than showing up in reports. Nip this in the bud by regular physical activity, a disciplined diet and sleep habits, and regular checkups. Once pathology manifests, you may need the crutches of external thyroid supplements. *Perhaps for life!*

Chalk, Clay and Cheese

Do you ever crave for abnormal stuff like mud, clay, chalk, paint, uncooked rice or even pencils, erasers and crayons? This is a medical condition called pica and could be the first sign of anemia. More serious conditions like obsessive disorders and autism need to be ruled out. After correcting any of the above, Cina 30/200c is an excellent remedy to reduce abnormal cravings. Though if you prefer chalk over cheese, enjoy at your own risk!

That Sprained Ankle

An innocuous ankle sprain may take as much or perhaps longer to heal than a fracture and needs equal care. While rest, elevation of the limb, bandaging and immobilization of the affected part are all mandatory, it would be worthwhile to take Arnica 30c twice daily for a week, followed by Rhus tox 30c for the next, both proven homeopathic remedies for early healing and pain reduction.

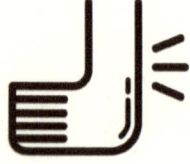

Waiting for the Burp

How do you know you have eaten enough? During a meal, a comfortable gentle fullness at the pit of your stomach, the desire to take the next helping not for hunger but for satiety and the stage until which you are still energetic not drowsy, are surefire signals to end your meal. *The burp is not mandatory!*

Unto Wellness

Strengthen your core immunity to maintain health even in polluted environments. Avoid crowded places, minimise vehicle usage, eat fresh, self-cooked food using local produce, drink filtered, boiled water, practise regular yoga to improve lung capacity, and spend a few minutes of the day in complete silence. Imbibing the best is the key to Wellness!

Nurture the Girl Child

Investing in the health of the adolescent girl child will equip her for physiological challenges in later years. A simple diet rich in proteins, iron and calcium, enough physical exercise with adequate sun exposure and access to basic sanitation is the least every girl is entitled to for, *on her health depends the health of the subsequent generation!*

Vitamin *Amla*

Amla (Indian gooseberry) has almost 15 times more Vitamin C than that of a lemon. However, its juice can cause acidity especially on an empty stomach. One suggestion – chop amla into small pieces and store in brine in the refrigerator. A few pieces with any of your meals will meet the daily vitamin C quota, *reduce the rate of infections and cut down doctor's vists too!*

Cleanliness Home-delivered

Most parasitic infestations, fungal infections and respiratory allergies can be prevented if rugs and carpets are vacuumed once a week and washed once a month, curtains washed once every 3 months, sofa covers, cushions, pillow covers once every two weeks, and bedsheets once a week in summer, twice a month in winter. Duvets, blankets should be dusted daily and washed regularly. Mops and dishcloths harbor maximum microbes; replacing them every month may cost a fraction of the cost incurred in treating those nagging worms or that unsightly fungal rash! *Cleanliness is the highway to health, wealth and godliness!*

Pray, for Wellness

Praying, even for a few minutes daily, boosts health by:

- reducing anxiety
- improving focus
- stabilising the heart rate
- lowering blood pressure.

Praying for someone else is even better as it involves compassion and release of feel-good hormones thus increasing immunity. *Note however, prayer is an adjuvant and not a substitute to medical treatment!*

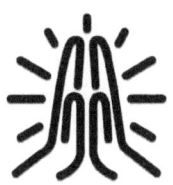

Do Your Homework

To avoid panic during an emergency, keep a copy of your complete health record, your family history in detail with a list of current medication, allergy to any drugs or food and all your contact details in a file for easy access. Also visit your GP regularly when you are well. *It makes it easier to treat you when you are sick!*

Whose Life is it Anyway?

In an ideal world, there would be no disease, only minor health aberrations; where there would only be natural mortality, no chronic, lingering disease. And, where doctors would be rewarded for keeping people healthy and penalized if they fell sick! Possible? Only if health becomes an individual responsibility and not that of a parent, spouse or government!

Strumming Fingers

Attention musicians, sports persons and weightlifters! The skin at the base of the thumb and other fingers may harden and get tender from repeated friction. Remedy: An application of Calendula ointment externally and Silicea 30c twice a day taken internally (available at the local homeopathy pharmacy) for two weeks *should help bring the music back into your routine!*

Mind your Fingers

Little children often get their fingers crushed between door hinges or window shutters. Apply cold compress immediately and give 2 pills each of Arnica and Hypericum 30c, in quick succession every 15 minutes, about 4 to 6 doses. There are no two ways about the efficacy of this combination: *helps reduce pain, inflammation and preserves the nail too!*

Phantom Pain

Of the various types of pains, the phantom pain is one of the most distressing. Often following amputation or a missing limb after an accident, phantom pain is a perception of pain, sometimes sharp, shooting or even burning, coming from the missing part of the body. Analgesics, anxiolytics and physiotherapy are the norm. However, it would be worthwhile prescribing Allium cepa 30c, an excellent, painless way to get rid of pain which is not there!

Plug That Leak

A persistent and nagging symptom, however minor, should never be left unaddressed. If ignored, it could lead to major health issues, sometimes life threatening! A leaking tap, a leaking nose or a leaking bladder ... get it corrected to avoid having dents in your finances and on your wellbeing! *For optimal health, financial and physical, plug that leak!*

Simple Fasting Rules

Fasting is not a weight loss program. Regular fasting actually trains one in self-restraint and delayed gratification, both qualities increasing mental tenacity. Start by fasting once a week on fluid and fruit. For total benefit, break your fast with a small, bland diet, and *not reward yourself with the goodies you perhaps missed!*

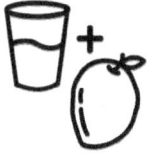

Razor Sharp

The summer humidity may cause itchy, painful eruptions in the beard area due to infected follicles – a highly contagious condition called barber's itch. The eruptions may ooze a sticky, yellowish pus on shaving. Washing often with soap and warm water, avoiding touching your face and taking homeopathic Graphites 30 should give relief within a week. *Guys, share your secrets, not your razor!*

Move on, Failure

Is failure a stepping stone to success? Not always. Recurring failure for the same reasons needs careful introspection, and if not accepted and worked on, can severely mar one's self confidence and motivation. A failure that is identified and dealt with persistence is not just a stepping stone but a sign of huge success coming one's way!

The Road Less Taken

When one travels to and sustains in unknown places with unknown language, it is actually therapeutic! Travelling to unfamiliar places helps in adapting and adjusting to a new environment. Learning a new language strengthens neural pathways making one more alert and agile! So, travel the path less travelled. For your own health!

Water Tales

When travelling to a place where water is hard, and you need to wash your hair, the best remedy is decantation. Fill a bucket with water, allow it to stand for 15 minutes (to allow hard minerals to settle) and scum off the upper layers leaving the last few mugs unused. This will improve softness of the water and may minimise the need for a hair conditioner too!

Starving a Fever

Feed a cold, starve a fever is a logical health advice. Eating well during a cold, mostly self-limiting, helps to build resistance. During a fever, the body's immune response is under stress to fight the infection. Eating minimum and simple with adequate hydration brings down the metabolism and the fever too. Do not force-feed a child with fever. *The pampering can happen during convalescence!*

Hair Where?

Regular exercise stimulates hair growth and excessive exercise may result in hair loss. Unless professionally monitored, an intense gym routine – pumping – is not recommended. Excess iron in the gym may increase testosterone causing male pattern baldness. Rather, opt for low intensity workouts coupled with brisk walking and yoga *to preserve your energy and your hair!*

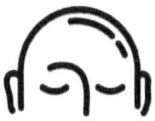

Only 99?

The curse of `99' may prove to be a hurdle in the route to mental well being. Persons who spend their vital years in a rat race, trying to convert 99 per cent to 100 per cent, linking perfection to happiness, seeking a perfect job, the perfect income, perfect relationships and perfect health parameters, end up suffering from anxiety, stress and ill health. Perfect health is not about perfect parameters. *It is about enjoying every step in the route to Wellness!*

Road Rage

Road rage is a psychological disorder in which a perfectly amiable and otherwise calm person turns violent on instigation. Mild road rage can be controlled with yoga, breath control and calm music. Extreme cases may need psychiatric help. Homeopathic Anacardium is an effective remedy to be taken on a homeopath's advice. A serious stressor for both sufferer and inflictor, *road rage must be addressed, not suppressed!*

Hearing in Style

Social isolation, dementia and decreased cognitive function in older people may not be related to neurological problems but to age-related hearing loss. With sophisticated and discreet hearing aids available, their use should be encouraged. Those little contraptions can go a long way in improving social communication in the elderly and *if worn with confidence, could become style statements too!*

A Pinch of Salt

When our grandmothers used a pinch of salt in confectionary and a bit of sugar in salted fritters, they were using solid scientific logic. Certain sensors move glucose to sweet taste cells in the presence of sodium, enhancing the sweetness and flavour without added sugar. Next time, if your glass of orange juice tastes sour, add no sugar, just that pinch of salt; *calorie count same, sweetness up!*

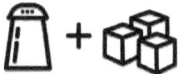

Shoulder Freeze

Frozen shoulder is nothing but an inflammation of the joint capsule causing intense pain, stiffness and restriction in movement. Homeopathy has excellent remedies to reduce inflammation and restore mobility. An effective remedy for chronic frozen shoulder is Causticum 30c. Taken for a couple of weeks along with appropriate physiotherapy may rid one of this nagging ailment.

Throw Away the Toxins

Management of diabetes and hypertension is the biggest step in preventing chronic kidney damage, a dangerous and silent killer. Plenty of water, fresh fruit and vegetables, low intake of salt and saturated fats and stress management are keys to renal health. A healthy kidney and a healthy nation will preserve the nutrients and throw out the toxins.

The responsibility is yours!

Your Doctor – Your Soldier

A doctor is a soldier guarding you from morbidity and mortality due to disease after years of sacrificing rest and recreation. As our armed forces deserve respect and honour so do the protectors of health and life. Caring for our doctors is actually safeguarding our own selves. A healthy doctor promotes better health and wellness. The soldier, the teacher and the doctor are special citizens of the nation. *They can take care of us only if we take care of them!*

The Unbeatable *Khichadi*

Replenishing the lost fluid and salts to maintain hydration is the main challenge when treating summer diarrhea. Most diarrheas are the body's defences to eliminate toxins and are mostly self-limiting. Give yourself 48 hours to recover during which stick to bland, soft diet, non-spicy, and non-fatty food. The rice lentil combo, the Indian *khichadi* is by far one of the best post diarrheal convalescent meals. *So nutritious, the normal and the constipated may have it too!*

Tough Back

Much of our back health depends on the choice of the mattress. A bad mattress can ruin the back and sleep. The right mattress must be firm, not hard ... soft, but not wobbly. Individual preference and adaptability can vary greatly; therefore, always buy the mattress after a trial of at least 48 hours. One secret though, the peaceful sleeper will sleep on rock and the insomniac will toss and turn. *The poor mattress will continue to be at the receiving end of the blame!*

Anna Purnabrahma

One should not live to eat and need not eat just to live. The ancient sages quoted *Anna purnabrahma* (*Anna* – food, *purnabrahma* – the celestial universe). Food at appropriate times, in appropriate composition and eaten with gratitude nourishes the body and soul and is an invocation to the Almighty! *It is the quest for daily bread that drives mankind, but greed that divides it!*

Think Abundance

Nature provides abundance, scarcity is manmade! Abundance is when one believes one has plenty, makes the best of what life has to offer and shares it generously with fellow human beings. Contentment is the secret of abundance. Surprisingly, the wealthiest may experience discontentment as nothing seems good enough, while the poor may experience contentment. *Practise abundance and see life getting simpler, happier and healthier!*

Springing the Pet Pack

Pet dogs and cats frequently suffer from cracks and fissures in their paws that may not respond to routine conventional measures. A few drops of Calendula 12c liquid mixed with Vaseline and applied gently to the paws and covered with soft gauze, along with homeopathic pills of Petroleum 30c, given twice a day, *is likely to get the spring back into your pet's feet!*

That Pain!

Pain difficult to bear and embarrassing to discuss – anal fissures and a few other ailments – can add misery and be prevented. Avoid constipation with enough water and fibre intake. A couple of prunes daily morning can ensure smooth bowel movement. Homeopathic remedy Acid nitric, taken thrice a day for a week, helps reduce pain and also heals the cuts. *Of course, surgery comes in when medicines fail!*

Strengthen That Shyness

Shyness, when extreme, may lead to social phobia and anxiety disorder. Try meeting new people, go on trips with strangers, and stay away from dominating people. Convert your shyness into strength. If not your tongue, use your eyes and ears to become keen observers and speak confidently at opportune moments. Take professional help, if necessary. *Do not shy away from seeing a counseler for your shyness!*

Herb Garden

Gardening is a superlative activity for the mind, body and soul, age no bar! No sprawling lawn? Even the window sill of your apartment will do. If every home grows these plants – holy basil (*tulsi*), aloe vera, lemon grass, Azadirachta (*neem*) and mint (*pudina*) – one gets food flavours, readymade home remedies and the best air purifiers; *all for just a little nurturing!*

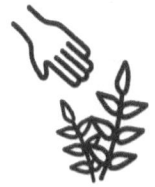

Greying Prematurely

One of the best ways to prevent premature greying of hair is to have an egg everyday. Apart from the essential minerals and proteins, the egg contains lecithin which strengthens and moistens the hair roots. For vegetarians, paneer, soya and corn may substitute the egg. However, stress management is the most vital factor in hair health. If that is a problem, take homeopathic Acid phos 30c, twice a day for a week and follow it with Lecithin 3x for a month to see the difference.

Thinning Eyebrows

Thinning of eyebrows is not a trivial condition – it can indicate serious diseases like autoimmune conditions, thyroid disorders, infections and chronic nutritional deficiencies. Diagnose and treat the root cause. Rubbing coconut oil gently over both brows daily will nourish the brows. If the eyes are the windows to the soul, the eyebrows are the checkposts of the eyes ... *preserve them with care!*

The Powerful Om

Chanting of a mantra, hymn or a word has immense health benefits. It strengthens the tongue, the vocal cords, glottis and trachea making them supple and improving respiratory capacity. Even a few minutes of regular chanting improves concentration and calms the mind. The mechanical vibration of the Om is *as scientific and as powerful as the electrical ohm!*

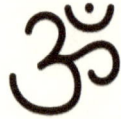

Stretch the Stiffness

Stretching is one of the simplest, easiest and most effective forms of exercise. Whether morning stiffness from arthritis or a midday slump, stretching one's limbs and back gradually, can instantly reduce muscle soreness and reduce dullness to make one feel energetic. Learning it under a trained physiotherapist is an excellent idea. For an active and healthy life, *stretch those muscles and never that argument!*

An Eye for the Eyes

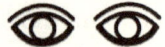

Kajal (kohl) is not just a cosmetic for eyes, it has immense health benefits too. Most commercially available *kajal* have lead sulphide – toxic and harmful to the eyes, to be especially avoided in babies. Organic *kajal* made from castor oil, camphor and activated charcoal moisturizes, protects and brightens the eyes. *Kajal* need not be banned, *it's the unhygienic application that needs to be corrected!*

Flying Ankles

Swollen ankles after a flight or long journey is likely to be due to venous insufficiency. Frequent movement, avoiding crossing legs and constant rotation of toes up and down and medially-laterally will keep the venous circulation going. Also, substituting salted snacks, soda, caffeinated drinks with plain water and fruit will maintain fluid electrolyte balance. For painful, swollen ankles following prolonged sitting, try Ledum 30c, thrice a day for a couple of days, *and you are ready to fly again!*

The 3 am Confidants

Do you have 3 am people in your life? Persons you can call up at any hour, who understand your anxieties, insecurities and secrets and stand by you no matter what, are the ones who contribute to your physical and mental health. Such bonds help reduce stress, provide a sense of belonging and boost confidence. *Lucky if you have 3 am friends; blessed, if you are one to someone!*

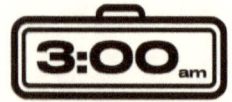

Healthy Investment

A good health portfolio is as necessary as the wealth portfolio. A balanced diet from early childhood with emphasis on key nutrients like iron, calcium and protein, along with daily exercise to build muscle strength and stamina – these are our fixed deposits, coming to our aid in times of illness. Meditation, cultivating hobbies and holding onto strong, healthy social relationships – they are our mutual funds. *No short term gains, value realized only after several years of investment!*

Blocked Ears?

Clogged ears can happen from congested sinuses, ear wax, blocked Eustachian tubes from infection or even exposure to sudden noise. Chronic sinusitis from repeated infection causing ear blockage responds effectively to Pulsatilla 200c, taken for a few days. *Disclaimer: No guarantee of recovering from exposure to shrieking from a nagging spouse!*

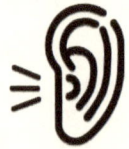

Raw *Kairi*

Switch to the younger sibling of the mango – the raw mango! Packed with as many nutrients as its riper version, it has a much higher content of Vit C, and certainly, lower sugar. Eaten raw, pickled, in curries, gravies, drinks and desserts, the *Kairi* (raw mango) enhances the flavour of every dish. Its high magnesium content ensures the smoothest movement of bowels possible … at least until the season lasts!

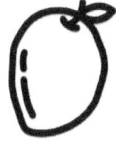

About the Author

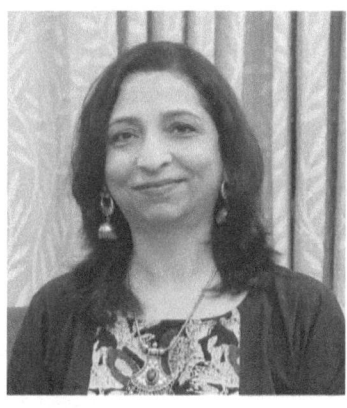

Dr. Sujata Naik, an M.D. in Homeopathy, has been running a hugely successful clinical practice in Mumbai, for more than three decades, with thousands of patients from India and abroad. She is also attached as an honorary homeopathic physician with the BKL Walawalkar Hospital, Dervan, in rural Maharashtra. Running a charitable OPD in this hospital, her work has seen significant impact at the grassroot level. She has succeeded in making inroads in areas where homeopathy has been previously unheard of. With her team of passionate homeopaths, Dr. Sujata Naik has been involved in several national and international research projects. Her work on the role of homeopathy in resistant fungal infections has been widely appreciated and has seen a host of awards at conferences at Cape Town, South Africa and Liverpool, UK, in 2018. She has also been awarded an honorary affiliation to the Faculty of Homeopathy, London, UK. A prolific writer, columnist and orator, Dr. Sujata Naik has been regularly invited as a speaker on various health forums. Her earlier book, The Wellness Shots has been listed by Notion Press in the bestsellers' category.

To know more about Dr. Sujata Naik's work, you can log onto www.drsujatanaik.com

Her social media posts can be followed at https://www.facebook.com/drsujatanaiksclinic/

www.ingramcontent.com/pod-product-compliance
Lightning Source LLC
Chambersburg PA
CBHW020916180526
45163CB00007B/2753